The lung guide to a healthy lung

A healthy lung

By

Peter A Godswill

Table of content

Introduction

A pair of healthy lungs is a marvel of biological engineering, silently working day in and day out to ensure the body receives a constant supply of oxygen and expels carbon dioxide. The respiratory system, comprising the lungs and a network of intricate airways, is not only essential for our survival but also plays a crucial role in maintaining overall health. This introductory section sets the stage for exploring the significance of healthy lung function and the practices that contribute to it.

In the pursuit of a holistic understanding of lung health, it is paramount to grasp the fundamental concepts of respiratory anatomy and physiology. The lungs, situated within the chest cavity, are composed of delicate tissues and a labyrinth of air sacs, blood vessels, and bronchioles. These structures work in harmonious synergy to facilitate the exchange of gases during respiration. Through inspiration, oxygen-rich air enters the lungs, where it diffuses into the bloodstream, nourishing cells throughout the body. Simultaneously, carbon dioxide, a metabolic waste product, is expelled from the bloodstream and exhaled from the body during expiration.

The Importance of lung health extends beyond mere biological functions. Healthy lungs play a vital role in maintaining energy levels, supporting physical activities, and ensuring mental clarity. They also act as a defense mechanism, filtering out harmful airborne particles and pathogens, thus protecting the body from potential infections. Moreover, optimal lung function contributes to maintaining a balanced pH level within the body, further emphasizing their role in overall homeostasis.

As the gateway between the body and the external environment, the respiratory system is exposed to a myriad of factors that can influence its well-being. From environmental pollutants and allergens to lifestyle choices such as smoking and poor nutrition, a multitude of factors can impact lung health. This introduction aims to ignite a deeper exploration into these factors and to shed light on the practices that can help maintain and promote healthy lungs.

In the subsequent sections of this guide, we will delve into the intricacies of respiratory anatomy, explore common lung-related issues, provide actionable tips for maintaining lung health, and discuss the importance of regular check-ups. By the end, we hope to equip you with knowledge that empowers you to make informed decisions about your lung health and well-being.

Chapter 1
What's a healthy lung

A healthy lung is a remarkable organ that functions efficiently to ensure the body receives a constant supply of oxygen while effectively expelling carbon dioxide, a waste product of metabolism. The definition of a healthy lung goes beyond the absence of disease; it encompasses optimal respiratory function, a well-maintained structure, and a robust defense against external threats.

At its core, a healthy lung boasts a high level of respiratory efficiency. This efficiency is marked by the lung's ability to efficiently exchange gases between the inhaled air and the bloodstream. Oxygen, essential for cellular metabolism and energy production, is diffused into the blood, while carbon dioxide, a byproduct of this process, is removed and exhaled. This exchange takes place across the intricate network of air sacs and capillaries within the lungs, facilitated by a thin barrier that allows gases to pass through easily.

In addition to efficient gas exchange, a healthy lung is characterized by its resilient structure. The lung's elastic tissues enable it to expand during inhalation and contract during exhalation, maintaining a steady rhythm of breathing. This flexibility ensures that the lung can adapt to various physical activities and conditions, supporting the body's oxygen demands even during exertion.

Furthermore, a healthy lung is equipped with an elaborate defense system. The airways are lined with tiny hair-like structures called cilia that move in coordinated waves, helping to trap and remove mucus along with any particles or pathogens that might have been inhaled. The immune cells within the lungs also play a pivotal role in identifying and neutralizing potential threats, such as bacteria or viruses.

Maintaining lung health requires a holistic approach, encompassing both preventive measures and lifestyle choices. Avoiding exposure to harmful environmental pollutants, such as tobacco smoke and industrial chemicals, is paramount. Regular physical activity promotes lung capacity and circulation, contributing to their overall vitality. Adequate hydration supports the thin mucus layer within the airways, aiding in the clearance of particles and irritants.

In essence, a healthy lung embodies a harmonious blend of efficient respiration, structural resilience, and vigilant defense mechanisms. Understanding the attributes of a healthy lung lays the foundation for recognizing deviations from this ideal state and taking proactive steps to safeguard and enhance one's respiratory well-being.

Lung health is a cornerstone of overall well-being, as these vital organs play a central role in sustaining life and maintaining the body's equilibrium. The significance of lung health extends far beyond their primary function of facilitating the exchange of oxygen and carbon dioxide. In this section, we delve into the multifaceted importance of maintaining healthy lungs.

First and foremost, optimal lung function is essential for the very survival of every cell in the body. Oxygen, obtained through respiration, is the fuel that powers cellular metabolism, enabling various biochemical reactions necessary for life. Without a steady supply of oxygen, cells would quickly cease to function, leading to a cascade of detrimental effects on organs and bodily systems.

Lung health is closely tied to cardiovascular health. The oxygen-rich blood pumped by the heart is distributed throughout the body, nourishing tissues and organs. Impaired lung function can lead to inadequate oxygenation of the blood, causing the heart to work

harder to compensate. Over time, this strain on the heart can contribute to cardiovascular diseases such as hypertension and heart failure.

Moreover, the lungs act as a natural filter, protecting the body from harmful environmental agents. Inhaling pollutants, allergens, and pathogens is an inevitable part of life, but healthy lungs are equipped with defense mechanisms to minimize their impact. Coughing, sneezing, and the secretion of mucus are all part of the lung's intricate defense system, which helps prevent these substances from entering the bloodstream and causing harm.

Lung health also has a profound impact on quality of life. Individuals with healthy lungs are better able to engage in physical activities, from brisk walks to strenuous workouts, without feeling short of breath.

Adequate lung capacity supports endurance, stamina, and overall vitality.

As society becomes increasingly aware of the long-term consequences of poor lung health, the importance of preventive measures and lifestyle choices becomes even more apparent. Avoiding exposure to smoke, pollutants, and other respiratory irritants is critical. Regular exercise not only supports lung function but also contributes to overall fitness. Equally important is

seeking medical attention at the first sign of respiratory distress, as early intervention can prevent minor issues from escalating into serious conditions.

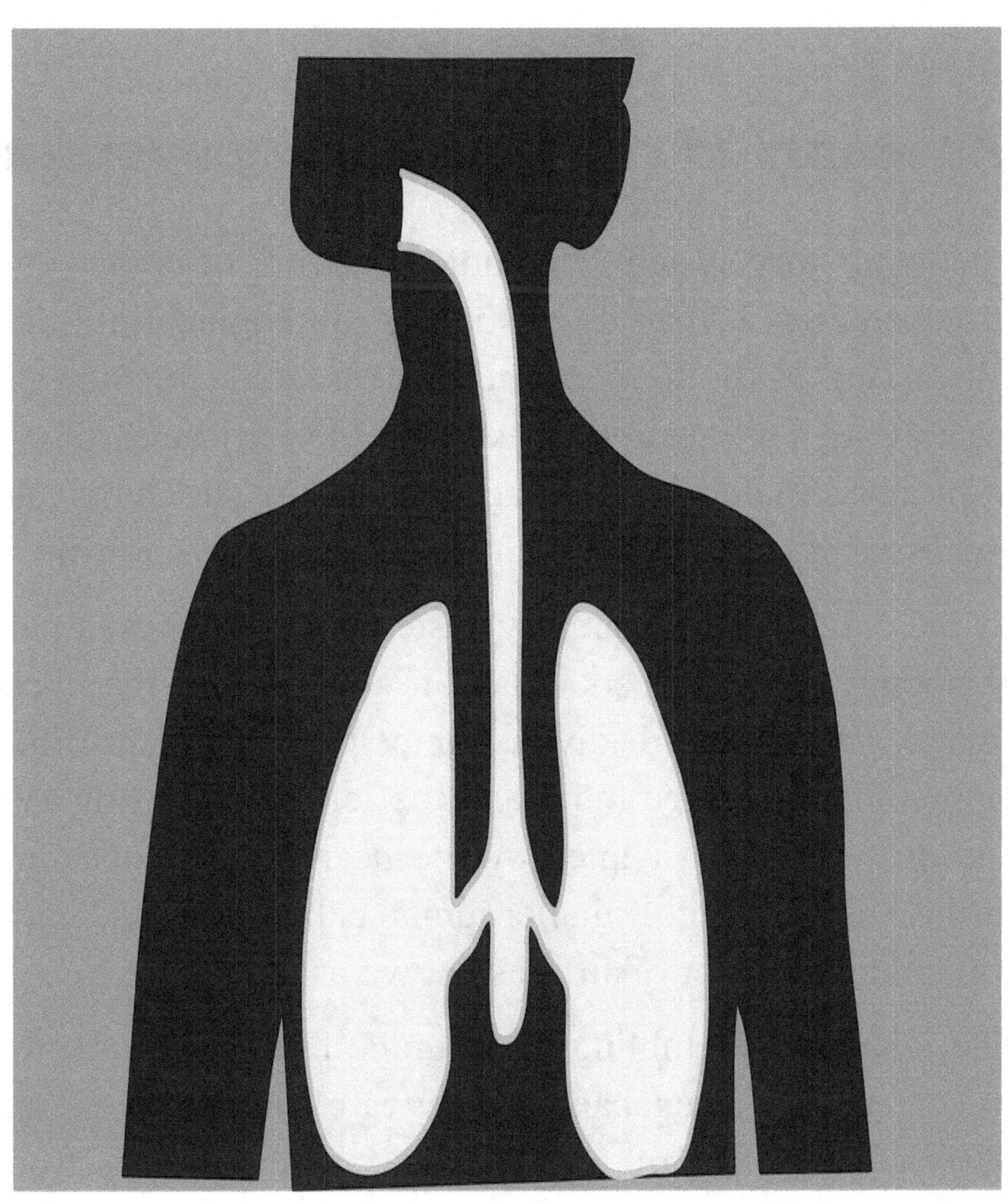

Chapter 2
Anatomy of the respiratory system

The respiratory system, a complex network of organs and structures, is a marvel of biological engineering that allows the body to perform the essential function of respiration. This section delves into the intricacies of the respiratory anatomy, shedding light on the structures and processes that enable the exchange of gases vital for life.

At the core of the respiratory system are the lungs, a pair of spongy, cone-shaped organs nestled within the chest cavity. The lungs are divided into lobes, with the right lung containing three lobes and the left lung housing two due to the space occupied by the heart. These lobes are further divided into smaller units called lobules, each containing a cluster of air sacs known as alveoli.

The alveoli, resembling tiny grape-like sacs, are the epicenter of gas exchange. They are enveloped by an intricate network of capillaries, where oxygen from inhaled air diffuses into the bloodstream, while carbon dioxide, a waste product, moves from the blood into the alveoli to be expelled during exhalation.

The process of respiration involves a series of movements within the chest cavity. During inhalation, the diaphragm, a dome-shaped muscle at the base of the lungs, contracts and flattens, causing the chest cavity to expand. This expansion lowers the air pressure within the lungs, allowing air to rush in and fill the alveoli. Exhalation, on the other hand, involves the relaxation of the diaphragm and the elastic recoil of lung tissues, expelling carbon dioxide-rich air from the alveoli.

The airways that lead to and from the lungs are equally crucial In this process. The trachea, commonly known as the windpipe, branches into smaller tubes called bronchi, which further divide into bronchioles. These progressively smaller airways are lined with cilia, tiny hair-like structures that constantly move in coordinated waves to clear mucus and trapped particles away from the lungs, preventing potential infections.

In conclusion, the anatomy of the respiratory system is a remarkable example of biological adaptation. From the lungs and alveoli responsible for gas exchange to the intricate network of airways designed to filter and clear the respiratory tract, each structure plays an indispensable role in enabling the fundamental process of respiration. Understanding the complexity of this system lays the foundation for appreciating the significance of maintaining its health and functionality.

Structure of the Lungs

At the heart of the respiratory system lie the lungs, two remarkable organs responsible for the exchange of gases between the body and the external environment. Situated within the chest cavity, the lungs are cushioned by the ribcage and separated by the heart.

The lungs consist of various lobes, with the right lung composed of three and the left lung comprising two. These lobes are further divided into smaller units called lobules. This division allows for efficient distribution of air and blood throughout the lungs, ensuring that no region is left without oxygenation. Each lobe and lobule houses an intricate network of air sacs known as alveoli.

Alveoli: These tiny, grape-like sacs are the primary sites of gas exchange. Enveloped by an extensive network of capillaries, alveoli provide an enormous surface area for the diffusion of gases. Oxygen, taken in during inhalation, passes from the alveoli into the bloodstream, while carbon dioxide, a waste product generated by cells, moves from the blood into the alveoli to be expelled during exhalation.

This exchange is driven by differences in partial pressures between the alveoli and the blood, a delicate balance that ensures efficient gas transfer.

Inhalation: When you inhale, the diaphragm contracts and flattens, and the ribcage expands. This movement increases the volume of the chest cavity, causing a decrease in air pressure within the lungs. As a result, outside air rushes in through the airways and into the alveoli, where oxygen molecules diffuse into the bloodstream.

Exhalation: Exhalation is a passive process in which the diaphragm relaxes and the ribcage returns to its original position due to elastic recoil. This reduces the volume of the chest cavity, leading to an increase in air pressure within the lungs. As a consequence, carbon dioxide-rich air is expelled from the alveoli and out of the body.

The respiratory system isn't solely responsible for gas exchange; it also plays a critical role in maintaining the body's acid-base balance. As cells metabolize nutrients, they produce carbon dioxide as a waste product. Carbon dioxide can form carbonic acid when dissolved in water, potentially leading to an acidic environment within the body. The respiratory system helps regulate this balance by adjusting the rate of breathing. Faster breathing expels more carbon dioxide, reducing its concentration and preventing excessive acidification.

Airways and Defense Mechanisms:

The airways leading to and from the lungs play a crucial role in filtering and protecting the respiratory system. The trachea, commonly known as the windpipe, branches into smaller tubes called bronchi, which continue to divide into even smaller bronchioles. These airways are lined with mucus-producing cells and cilia, tiny hair-like structures that constantly move in coordinated waves.

Mucus traps particles, pathogens, and other irritants that may have been inhaled. The cilia then move in coordinated motions to propel the mucus and trapped debris away from the lungs and toward the throat, where it can be swallowed or expelled through coughing or sneezing. This system serves as a natural defense mechanism, preventing potentially harmful substances from reaching the delicate alveoli and causing infections or irritation.

Conclusion:

The intricate anatomy of the respiratory system reflects its crucial role in sustaining life. From the lungs' alveoli, where gas exchange takes place, to the airways' cilia that protect against airborne threats, each structure plays a unique and essential role in ensuring efficient respiration. Understanding this anatomy provides insights into the mechanisms behind breathing, gas exchange, and the body's ability to maintain its acid-base balance. As we continue to explore the respiratory system's intricacies, we gain a deeper appreciation for its complexity and the vital role it plays in supporting human life.

Chapter 3
Common respiratory issues

The respiratory system, while marvelously designed, is not immune to challenges. This section delves into the diverse array of common respiratory issues that can impact lung health, exploring their causes, symptoms, and potential management strategies.

Overview of Lung Diseases:

Lung diseases encompass a broad spectrum of conditions that affect the respiratory system's structure and function. From infections and inflammations to chronic conditions and genetic disorders, these ailments can significantly impact a person's quality of life and overall well-being.

Respiratory Infections: Infections of the respiratory tract are among the most prevalent lung issues. Common colds, caused by various viruses, often lead to symptoms like coughing, sneezing, and congestion. Influenza, or the flu, is another viral infection that can cause severe respiratory symptoms and even lead to complications. Bacterial infections like pneumonia affect the air sacs in the lungs, causing inflammation and potentially impairing gas exchange.

Chronic Obstructive Pulmonary Disease (COPD): COPD is a group of progressive lung diseases, including emphysema and chronic bronchitis. Long-term exposure to irritants, particularly cigarette smoke, is a leading cause of COPD. These diseases cause obstruction of airflow, resulting in symptoms such as shortness of breath, chronic cough, and wheezing.

Asthma: Asthma is characterized by recurrent episodes of airflow obstruction, often triggered by allergens or irritants. During an asthma attack, the airways become inflamed and constricted, leading to difficulty breathing, chest tightness, and wheezing. While there is no cure for asthma, it can be managed through medications and lifestyle changes.

Lung Cancer: Lung cancer is a serious condition characterized by the uncontrolled growth of abnormal cells in the lungs. It is strongly associated with smoking but can also occur in non-smokers due to other risk factors such as exposure to secondhand smoke or environmental pollutants. Early detection and treatment are crucial for improving outcomes.

Interstitial Lung Diseases: These disorders affect the lung's interstitium, the tissue that supports the alveoli. Conditions like pulmonary fibrosis involve scarring of the interstitium, leading to reduced lung function and breathlessness.

Causes and Risk Factors:

Understanding the causes and risk factors of common respiratory issues is vital for prevention, early detection, and management.

Smoking: Smoking is perhaps the most significant risk factor for a wide range of lung diseases. It damages the airways, impairs lung function, and increases the likelihood of infections and cancer.

Environmental Factors: Exposure to environmental pollutants such as air pollutants, dust, and chemicals can contribute to respiratory issues. Occupational hazards like asbestos exposure can also lead to lung disease.

Genetic Factors: Some respiratory conditions, like cystic fibrosis, have a genetic component. Individuals with a family history of lung diseases may be at a higher risk.

Allergens: Allergens like pollen, mold, and pet dander can trigger respiratory symptoms, particularly in individuals with allergies or asthma.

Age and Gender: Age can increase susceptibility to certain lung diseases, with conditions like COPD being more common in older individuals. Gender can also play a role, as women tend to have smaller airways, making them more vulnerable to respiratory issues.

Prevention and Management:

While some respiratory issues may be unavoidable due to genetic factors or environmental exposures, many can be prevented or managed through proactive measures.

Lifestyle Choices: Quitting smoking and avoiding exposure to secondhand smoke are paramount for lung health. Maintaining a healthy diet and engaging in regular exercise can also support lung function.

Environmental Awareness: Minimizing exposure to air pollutants, indoor allergens, and occupational hazards can significantly reduce the risk of respiratory issues.

Vaccinations: Immunizations against infections like influenza and pneumonia are crucial, particularly for individuals with compromised lung health.

Early Detection: Regular check-ups and lung function tests can aid in the early detection of respiratory issues, allowing for timely intervention and management.

Medications and Treatments: Depending on the specific condition, various medications and treatments are available. These may include bronchodilators, anti-inflammatory drugs, oxygen therapy, and pulmonary rehabilitation.

Conclusion: Common respiratory issues encompass a diverse range of conditions that can impact lung health and overall well-being. From infections and chronic diseases to genetic predispositions, these challenges underline the importance of maintaining lung health through preventive measures, early detection, and appropriate management strategies. By understanding the causes, symptoms, and potential risks associated with these conditions, individuals can take proactive steps to safeguard their respiratory health and lead a fulfilling and active life.

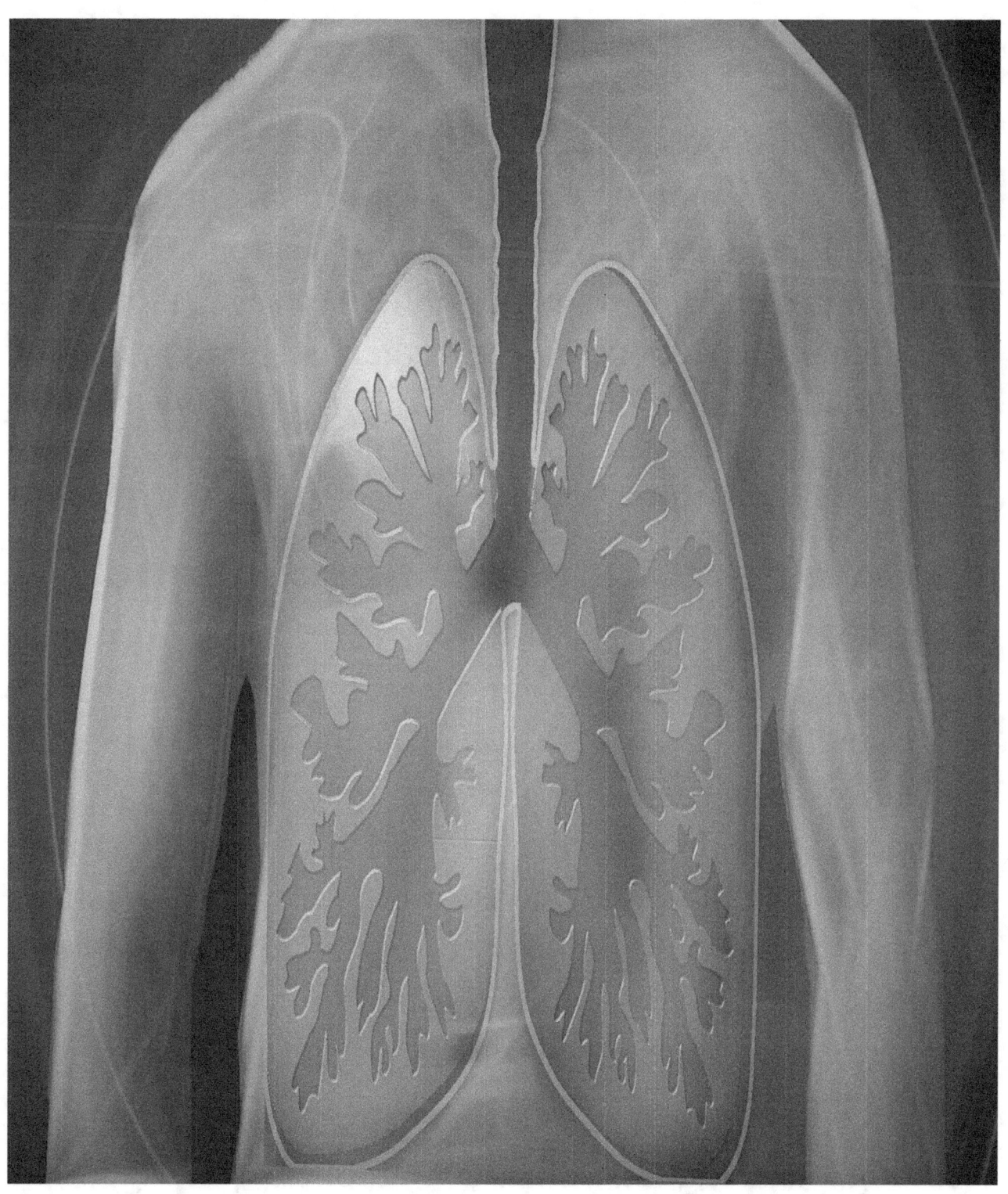

Chapter 4

Tips for maintaining a healthy lung

Maintaining healthy lungs is essential for overall well-being and quality of life. This section explores a comprehensive set of strategies and practices that can help individuals proactively care for their respiratory health, from avoiding harmful habits to adopting lifestyle choices that promote optimal lung function.

Avoiding Smoking and Secondhand Smoke

Tobacco smoke, whether from direct smoking or exposure to secondhand smoke, is one of the most significant threats to lung health. It contains thousands of harmful chemicals that damage the delicate lung tissues, impair the cilia's function, and increase the risk of lung cancer, chronic obstructive pulmonary disease (COPD), and other respiratory issues. Avoiding smoking and minimizing exposure to secondhand smoke is crucial for maintaining healthy lungs.

Quitting Smoking. If you are a smoker, quitting is the most impactful step you can take to improve lung health. The benefits of quitting begin almost immediately, with improved lung function, reduced risk of infections, and a decreased likelihood of developing serious respiratory diseases.

Creating Smoke-Free Environments: Creating a smoke-free environment is equally important. If you live with or around smokers, encourage them to quit or ask them to smoke outside to minimize your exposure to secondhand smoke.

Indoor Air Quality and Lung Health:

The air quality within your home and workplace can significantly impact your lung health. Indoor pollutants, including dust, mold, allergens, and chemicals, can exacerbate respiratory symptoms and increase the risk of lung diseases. Taking steps to improve indoor air quality is essential for maintaining healthy lungs.

Adequate Ventilation: Proper ventilation helps reduce indoor air pollutants. Ensure that your living and working spaces are well-ventilated by opening windows and using exhaust fans when needed.

Regular Cleaning: Regular cleaning, dusting, and vacuuming help minimize the accumulation of dust, pollen, and allergens. Using air purifiers with HEPA filters can further improve air quality.

Controlling Humidity: Maintaining appropriate humidity levels (around 30-50%) can help prevent the growth of mold and reduce the risk of respiratory issues.

Exercise and Lung Function:

Regular physical activity has a positive impact on lung health and function. Exercise helps improve lung capacity, strengthens respiratory muscles, and enhances oxygen exchange efficiency. Engaging in regular cardiovascular exercises, such as brisk walking, jogging, swimming, or cycling, can contribute to maintaining healthy lungs.

Aerobic Exercises: Aerobic activities increase lung capacity and cardiovascular fitness. Aim for at least 150 minutes of moderate-intensity aerobic exercise each week.

Breathing Exercises: Certain breathing exercises, like pursed-lip breathing and diaphragmatic breathing, can enhance lung function and help manage breathlessness.

Strength Training: Incorporating strength training exercises, which target various muscle groups, can also support lung health by improving overall fitness.

Proper Nutrition for Lung Health:

Diet plays a significant role in supporting lung health by providing essential nutrients that help maintain the integrity of lung tissues, support the immune system, and reduce inflammation.

Antioxidant-Rich Foods: Antioxidants, found in fruits and vegetables like berries, citrus fruits, spinach, and bell peppers, help protect lung tissues from oxidative stress and damage.

Omega-3 Fatty Acids: Sources of omega-3 fatty acids, like fatty fish (salmon, mackerel), flaxseeds, and walnuts, have anti-inflammatory properties that can benefit lung health.

Vitamin D: Adequate vitamin D levels are associated with better lung function. Some sources of vitamin D include fatty fish, fortified dairy products, and sunlight exposure.

Hydration: Staying hydrated helps maintain the thin layer of mucus in the airways, supporting the body's natural defense mechanism against irritants and pathogens.

Respiratory Hygiene Practices:

Practicing good respiratory hygiene is essential for preventing the spread of infections and maintaining lung health.

Hand Hygiene: Regularly washing hands with soap and water for at least 20 seconds helps prevent the transmission of viruses and bacteria.

Cough Etiquette: Cover your mouth and nose with a tissue or your elbow when coughing or sneezing to prevent the spread of respiratory droplets.

Avoiding Close Contact: During periods of illness or outbreaks, avoiding close contact with individuals who are sick can reduce the risk of infection.

Vaccinations: Immunizations against influenza and pneumonia can provide additional protection against respiratory infections.

Caring for your lung health involves a holistic approach that encompasses healthy habits, proactive measures, and a conscious effort to minimize risk factors. From avoiding smoking and secondhand smoke to adopting regular exercise, maintaining a balanced diet, and practicing respiratory hygiene, each strategy contributes to the overall well-being of your lungs. By implementing these tips and making conscious choices that prioritize lung health, you can enjoy a life marked by vitality, endurance, and a reduced risk of respiratory issues.

Conclusion:

In conclusion, the journey through the world of lung health has revealed the intricate interplay of anatomy, function, and practices that contribute to overall well-being. Healthy lungs, essential for sustaining life, are not just passive organs but dynamic systems that require care and attention.

Throughout this exploration, we've learned that a healthy lung is characterized by efficient gas exchange, resilient structure, and vigilant defense mechanisms. From the alveoli's delicate dance of oxygen and carbon dioxide to the airways' protective cilia, every component plays a vital role in maintaining optimal respiratory function.

Recognizing the importance of lung health extends beyond the realm of biology. Healthy lungs enable us to engage in physical activities with vigor, support our mental clarity, and protect us from harmful environmental agents. They contribute to the equilibrium of the body's pH levels and the overall homeostasis that keeps us functioning optimally.

However, the road to maintaining healthy lungs is not without challenges. Respiratory issues, ranging from infections and allergies to chronic diseases and genetic predispositions, remind us of the need for vigilance and care. Avoiding smoking, secondhand smoke, and environmental pollutants is essential for preventing damage and maintaining lung vitality. Engaging in regular exercise, prioritizing proper nutrition, and practicing good respiratory hygiene further fortify our lung health defenses.

As we close this exploration, let us reflect on the significance of lung health in our lives. It's a journey marked by choices, awareness, and an ongoing commitment to nurturing our lungs' well-being. By understanding the factors that impact lung health, adopting preventive measures, and making informed choices, we empower ourselves to lead lives rich in vitality, energy, and the freedom to breathe deeply and fully. May the knowledge gained within these pages inspire you to prioritize your lung health, enriching your journey through wellness and vitality.

Nourishing Lung Health: A Cookbook for Respiratory Wellness

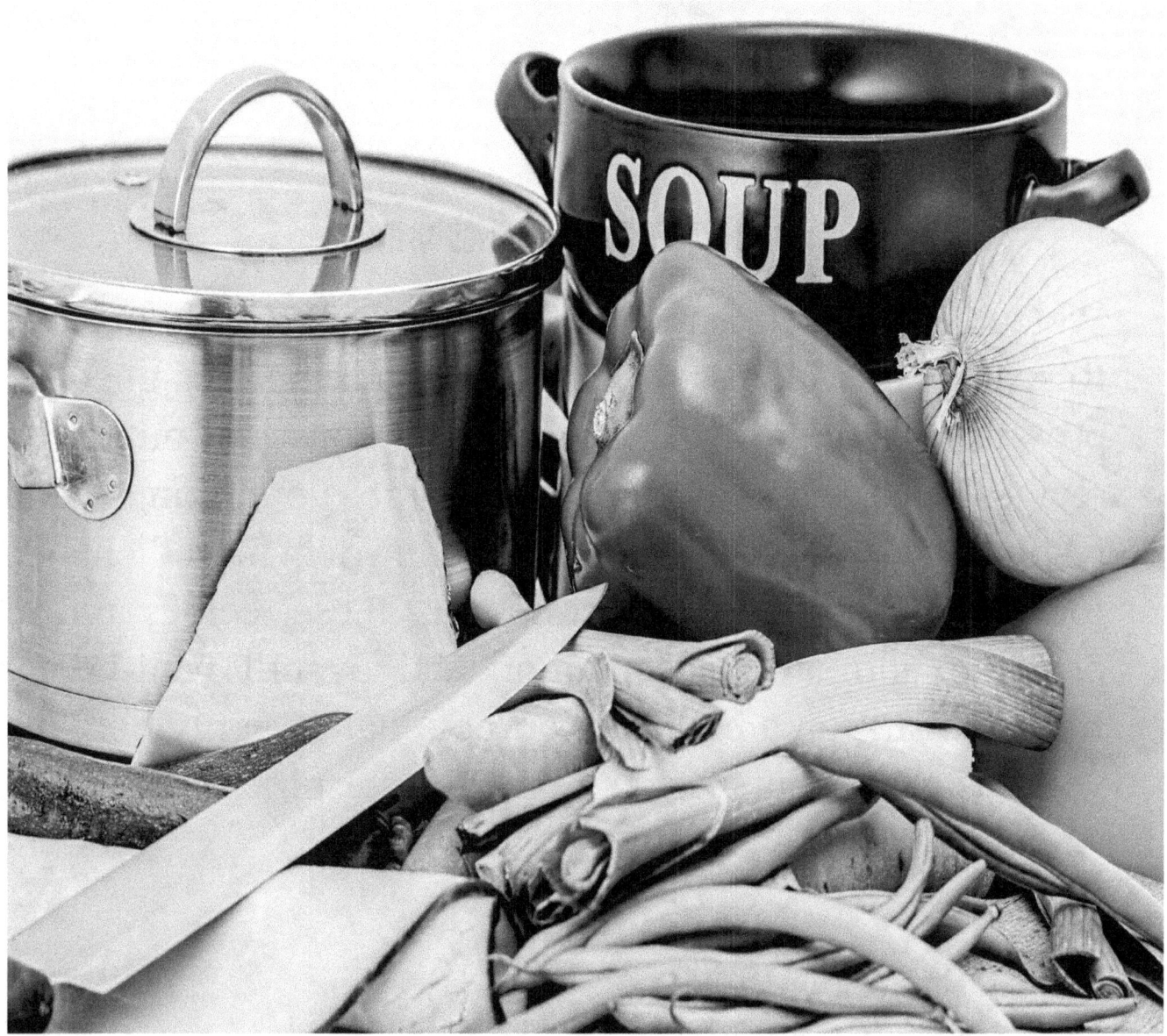

Introduction:

Welcome to "Nourishing Lung Health: A Cookbook for Respiratory Wellness." This cookbook is designed to provide you with a collection of delicious and nutritious recipes that support the health of your lungs and respiratory system. From antioxidant-rich ingredients to foods rich in vitamins and minerals, these recipes aim to promote optimal lung function and overall well-being. Let's embark on a culinary journey that not only delights your taste buds but also supports your respiratory health.

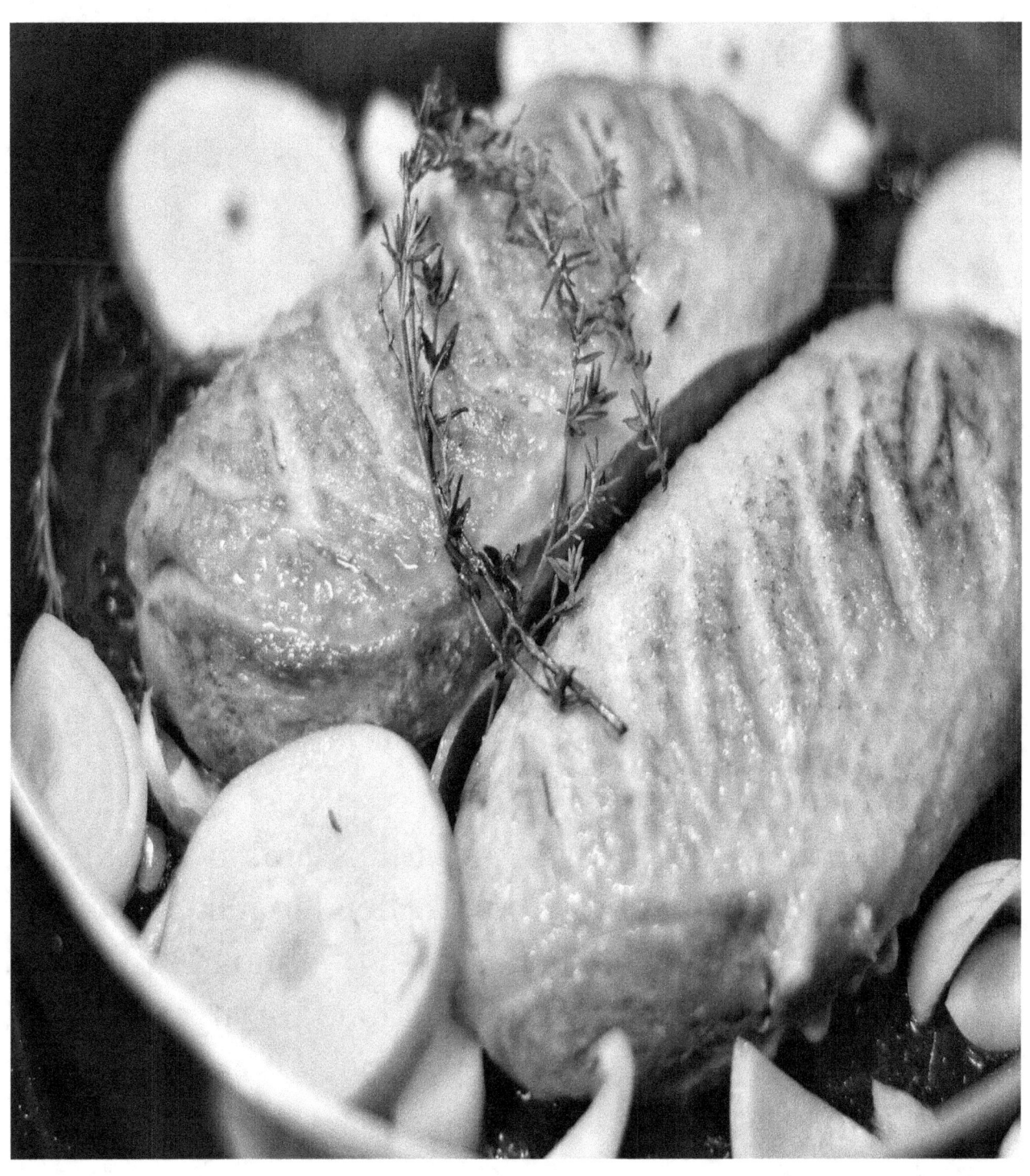

Chapter 5: Fresh Start Breakfasts

1. Green Smoothie Bowl

2. Oatmeal with Berries and Nuts

3. Avocado Toast with Poached Egg

Chapter 1: Fresh Start Breakfasts

In "Nourishing Lung Health: A Cookbook for Respiratory Wellness," we believe that starting your day with a nutrient-packed breakfast sets the tone for overall well-being. This chapter introduces you to a variety of delicious and lung-friendly breakfast options that combine essential nutrients to fuel your body and support your respiratory health.

1. Green Smoothie Bowl:

Begin your day with a burst of antioxidants by indulging in a vibrant green smoothie bowl. Blend together spinach, kale, banana, pineapple, and a splash of almond milk for a refreshing and nutrient-rich concoction. Top it with sliced berries, chia seeds, and a drizzle of honey for added flavor and texture.

2. Oatmeal with Berries and Nuts:

Oats are an excellent source of soluble fiber that can contribute to lung health. Prepare a comforting bowl of oatmeal using rolled oats and water or your preferred milk. Top it with a handful of mixed berries, chopped nuts, and a sprinkle of cinnamon for a delightful combination of flavors and textures.

3. Avocado Toast with Poached Egg:

Avocado is packed with healthy fats that can support lung function. Spread mashed avocado on whole grain toast and top it with a perfectly poached egg. Season with a pinch of salt, pepper, and a sprinkle of red pepper flakes for a satisfying and protein-rich breakfast.

Each of these breakfast options not only provides a boost of energy to start your day but also includes ingredients that contribute to lung health. By incorporating a variety of fruits, vegetables, and whole grains, you'll be nourishing your body while supporting your respiratory system. Stay tuned as we explore more recipes that promote lung wellness throughout this cookbook.

Chapter 6: Vibrant Salads for Lunch

Chapter 2: Vibrant Salads for Lunch

In this chapter of "Nourishing Lung Health: A Cookbook for Respiratory Wellness," we shift our focus to invigorating salads that are not only packed with flavor but also rich in nutrients to support your lung health. Salads are a fantastic way to incorporate a variety of vegetables, fruits, lean proteins, and whole grains into your diet, providing you with a well-rounded and nourishing meal.

1. Spinach and Berry Salad with Grilled Chicken:

Combine fresh spinach leaves, juicy berries, and slices of grilled chicken for a satisfying and antioxidant-rich salad. Add a sprinkle of feta cheese and a handful of toasted almonds for a delightful crunch. Drizzle with a balsamic vinaigrette made from olive oil, balsamic vinegar, Dijon mustard, and a touch of honey.

Citrus Kale Salad with Walnuts and Feta:

Kale is known for its high vitamin and mineral content, making it an excellent choice for supporting lung health. Massage chopped kale leaves with a zesty citrus vinaigrette, then top the salad with segments of orange, crumbled feta cheese, and toasted walnuts for added texture and flavor.

2. Quinoa Salad with Roasted Vegetables:

Quinoa, a protein-rich grain, takes center stage in this hearty salad. Roast a colorful array of vegetables like bell peppers, zucchini, and cherry tomatoes, and mix them with cooked quinoa. Drizzle with a lemon herb dressing made from lemon juice, olive oil, minced garlic, and fresh herbs like basil and parsley.

These salad recipes are designed to keep you feeling satisfied and energized throughout your day, all while providing your body with essential nutrients for optimal lung health. By incorporating a variety of ingredients and flavors, you'll find that salads can be anything but boring and are a delightful way to support your respiratory wellness. Stay tuned as we dive into more chapters filled with lung-loving recipes!

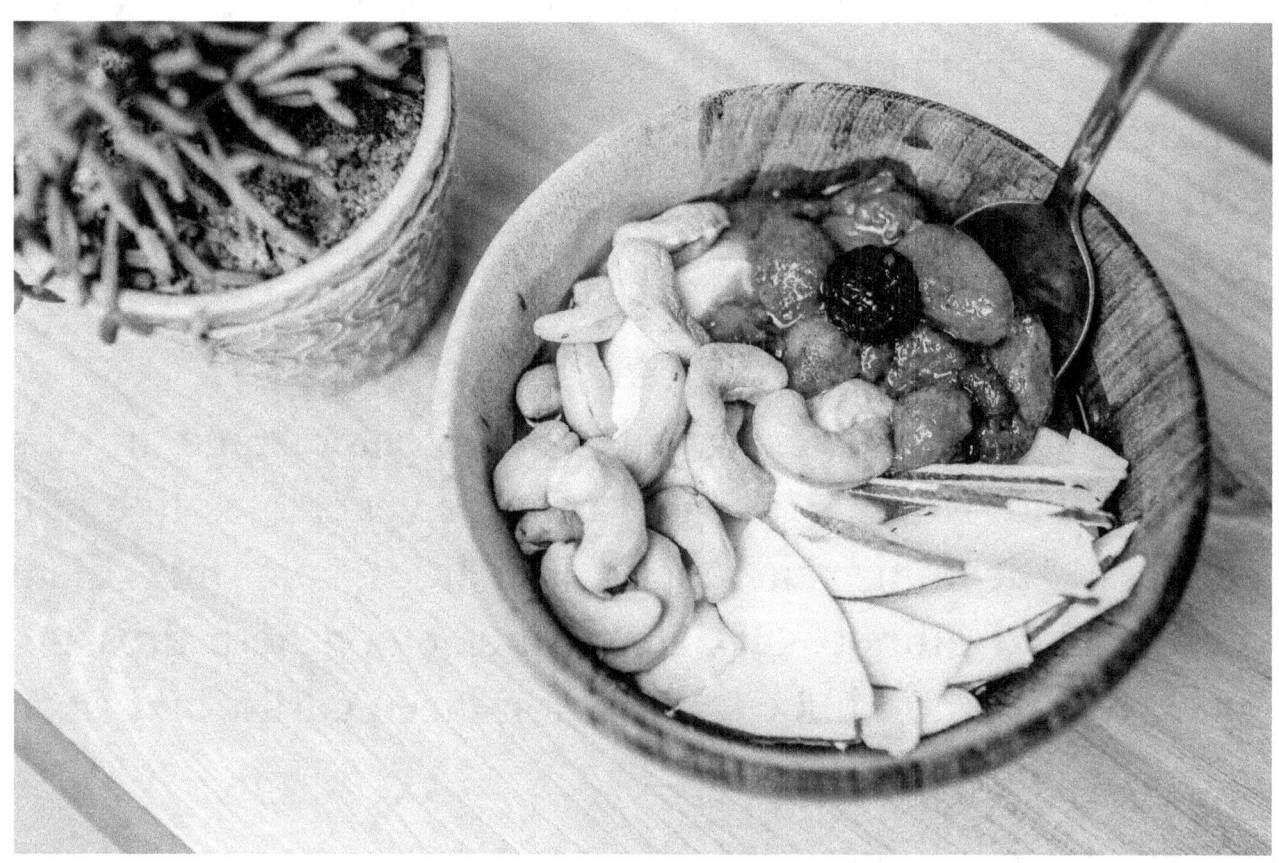

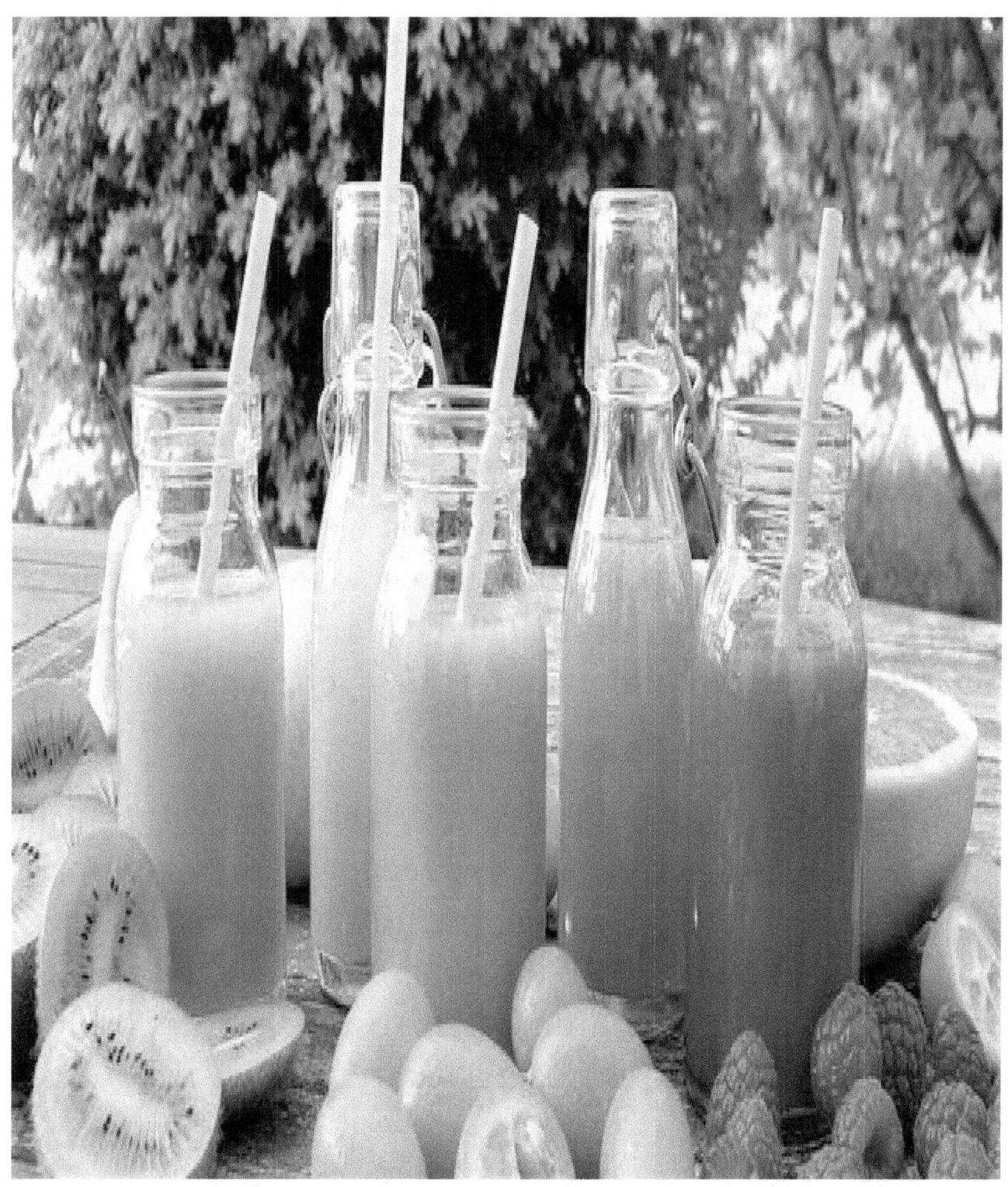

Chapter 7: Wholesome Soups and Stews

7. Lentil and Vegetable Soup

8. Chicken and Ginger Congee

9. Minestrone with Whole Grain Pasta

Welcome to the heartwarming chapter of "Nourishing Lung Health: A Cookbook for Respiratory Wellness" dedicated to wholesome soups and stews. These comforting and flavorful dishes not only provide comfort on a chilly day but also offer a rich source of nutrients to support your respiratory health. Let's explore the recipes that will warm your soul and nourish your lungs.

3. Lentil and Vegetable Soup:

Lentils are a fantastic source of plant-based protein and fiber, making them an excellent addition to any lung-friendly diet. Combine lentils with an array of colorful vegetables like carrots, celery, and spinach. Flavor the soup with aromatic herbs and spices, such as cumin and turmeric, to create a hearty and flavorful dish.

4 Chicken and Ginger Congee:

Congee, a rice porridge, is a soothing and easily digestible dish that can provide comfort and nutrients. Simmer rice with ginger and shredded chicken until it reaches a creamy consistency. The ginger not only adds warmth but also possesses anti-inflammatory properties that can benefit respiratory health.

4. Minestrone with Whole Grain Pasta:

Minestrone is a classic Italian soup brimming with a variety of vegetables and beans. Boost the nutritional content by using whole grain pasta for added fiber and nutrients. With ingredients like tomatoes, beans, and leafy greens, this soup offers a medley of flavors and nutrients that can support your lung wellness.

These soup and stew recipes are a perfect way to incorporate a variety of ingredients into your diet while enjoying nourishing and comforting meals. The warmth and depth of flavors in these dishes make them a delightful addition to your lung health journey. As we continue through this cookbook, get ready to explore more recipes that contribute to your overall well-being.

Chapter 8: Nutrient-Rich Dinners

10. Baked Salmon with Lemon and Dill

11. Tofu Stir-Fry with Broccoli and Bell Peppers

12. Turkey Meatballs with Zucchini Noodles

Welcome to the flavorful world of nutrient-rich dinners in "Nourishing Lung Health: A Cookbook for Respiratory Wellness." This chapter is dedicated to providing you with a range of satisfying dinner options that incorporate lean proteins, vibrant vegetables, and wholesome grains to support your lung health. Let's delve into these delicious and nourishing recipes.

5. Baked Salmon with Lemon and Dill:

Salmon is a fantastic source of omega-3 fatty acids, which are known to have anti-inflammatory properties that can benefit respiratory health. Marinate salmon fillets with lemon, dill, and a touch of olive oil, then bake until perfectly flaky. Serve alongside steamed asparagus and quinoa for a complete and wholesome meal.

6. Tofu Stir-Fry with Broccoli and Bell Peppers:

Tofu is a plant-based protein that can be transformed into a delectable stir-fry. Sauté cubed tofu with an array of colorful vegetables like broccoli, bell peppers, and snap peas. Create a savory stir-fry sauce using low-sodium soy sauce, ginger, garlic, and a drizzle of sesame oil. Serve over brown rice or whole wheat noodles.

7. Turkey Meatballs with Zucchini Noodles:

Lean ground turkey is the star of this recipe, providing a lean source of protein to fuel your body. Form turkey meatballs seasoned with herbs and spices, then bake until golden. Create zucchini noodles using a spiralizer and sauté them lightly. Top the noodles with the turkey meatballs and a simple tomato sauce for a light and satisfying dinner.

These nutrient-rich dinner recipes not only satisfy your taste buds but also contribute to your lung health journey. By incorporating a variety of proteins, vegetables, and grains, you're providing your body with the essential nutrients it needs to function at its best. As we continue through this cookbook, you'll discover more recipes designed to support your respiratory wellness.

Chapter 9: Sides and Snacks

13. Roasted Garlic Hummus with Veggie Sticks

14. Kale Chips with Sea Salt

15. Mixed Nuts and Seeds Trail Mix

Welcome to the versatile chapter of "Nourishing Lung Health: A Cookbook for Respiratory Wellness." In this section, we explore a variety of sides and snacks that not only make excellent accompaniments to your meals but also contribute to your lung health journey. These options are designed to provide a balance of flavors and nutrients to keep you satisfied throughout the day.

8. Roasted Garlic Hummus with Veggie Sticks:

Hummus is a nutrient-packed dip that can be enjoyed with an array of colorful vegetable sticks. Blend cooked chickpeas, tahini, roasted garlic, lemon juice, and olive oil to create a creamy and flavorful hummus. Serve it alongside carrot, celery, and bell pepper sticks for a crunchy and satisfying snack.

9. Kale Chips with Sea Salt:

Kale chips are a nutritious and crunchy alternative to traditional potato chips. Tear kale leaves into bite-sized pieces, toss them with a drizzle of olive oil and a pinch of sea salt, then bake until they turn crispy. These kale chips offer a satisfying crunch while providing a dose of vitamins and minerals.

10. Mixed Nuts and Seeds Trail Mix:

Nuts and seeds are rich in healthy fats, protein, and essential nutrients that support your lung health. Create a customized trail mix by combining almonds, walnuts, pumpkin seeds, and dried berries. Portion them into small servings for a convenient and satisfying snack on the go.

These sides and snacks offer a variety of textures and flavors to keep your taste buds engaged while nourishing your body. Whether you're looking for a quick pick-me-up or a light accompaniment to your main meals, these options provide a balance of nutrients that contribute to your overall respiratory wellness. Stay tuned as we delve into more chapters filled with lung-loving recipes!

Chapter 10: Drinks for Lung Support

16. Herbal Tea Blend for Respiratory Health

17. Fresh Ginger and Turmeric Infused Water

18. Green Smoothie with Spinach and Pineapple

In "Nourishing Lung Health: A Cookbook for Respiratory Wellness," we understand that what you drink is just as important as what you eat. This chapter introduces you to a selection of beverages designed to provide hydration, nourishment, and respiratory support. Let's explore the refreshing and lung-friendly drink options that will complement your meals and enhance your well-being.

11. Herbal Tea Blend for Respiratory Health:

Sip on a soothing cup of herbal tea that promotes lung health. Combine ingredients like thyme, eucalyptus, and licorice root for a blend that supports respiratory wellness. These herbs are known for their potential to ease congestion and provide comfort when you're feeling under the weather.

12. Fresh Ginger and Turmeric Infused Water:

Ginger and turmeric are potent anti-inflammatory ingredients that can benefit your lungs. Create an infused water by adding thin slices of fresh ginger and turmeric to a pitcher of water. Let the flavors infuse for a few hours, then enjoy a refreshing and aromatic drink that provides a subtle kick of warmth and wellness.

13. Green Smoothie with Spinach and Pineapple:

Green smoothies are a fantastic way to incorporate a variety of nutrients into your diet. Blend together fresh spinach, pineapple, banana, and a splash of coconut water for a hydrating and nutrient-packed drink. The spinach adds a dose of vitamins and minerals that can support your respiratory health.

These drink recipes offer a range of flavors and benefits that contribute to your overall lung wellness. Whether you're seeking comfort, hydration, or a boost of nutrients, these beverages are a delicious way to complement your meals and take a step towards supporting your respiratory system. As we continue through this cookbook, get ready to explore more recipes that align with your health goals.

Chapter 11: Sweet Treats with Benefits

19. Blueberry Chia Seed Pudding

20. Dark Chocolate Covered Almonds

21. Greek Yogurt Parfait with Honey and Berries

Welcome to the delectable world of sweet treats that align with your lung health journey in "Nourishing Lung Health: A Cookbook for Respiratory Wellness." In this chapter, we'll introduce you to a collection of desserts that not only satisfy your sweet tooth but also provide nutritional value to support your overall well-being.

14. Blueberry Chia Seed Pudding:

Chia seeds are packed with omega-3 fatty acids and fiber, making them a wonderful addition to your diet. Create a creamy chia seed pudding by combining chia seeds with almond milk and a touch of honey. Layer the pudding with fresh blueberries for a delightful and antioxidant-rich dessert.

15. Dark Chocolate Covered Almonds:

Dark chocolate contains antioxidants and may have anti-inflammatory properties that can benefit your lungs. Dip almonds in melted dark chocolate and let them cool until the chocolate hardens. Enjoy these dark chocolate-covered almonds as a satisfying and guilt-free indulgence.

16. Greek Yogurt Parfait with Honey and Berries:

Greek yogurt is a protein-packed base for a wholesome and delightful parfait. Layer Greek yogurt with a drizzle of honey, mixed berries, and a sprinkle of granola. This parfait provides a balance of textures and flavors while offering a dose of probiotics that can contribute to your digestive and respiratory wellness.

These sweet treats with benefits are designed to show that desserts can be enjoyed as part of a balanced and lung-friendly diet. By incorporating ingredients rich in antioxidants and nutrients, you can indulge in these treats while still supporting your respiratory health goals. As we conclude this cookbook, we hope you've discovered a variety of recipes that inspire you to make mindful food choices and embark on a journey of well-being.

Conclusion:

We hope this cookbook inspires you to make mindful food choices that contribute to the well-being of your lungs. Remember that a balanced diet rich in nutrients can positively impact your respiratory health. Enjoy the journey of exploring these recipes, and may your meals be both nourishing and delicious. Breathe easy and live well!

www.ingramcontent.com/pod-product-compliance
Lightning Source LLC
Chambersburg PA
CBHW082229290526
45794CB00009B/3727